Amoxicillin

The Ultimate Guide to Deal with Pneumonia, Respiratory Tract Infections, Urinary Tract Infections, Otitis Media, Tooth Infections and Many More Using Antibiotics

Paul Sullivan

PUBLISHED BY: Paul Sullivan

First Print 2024

Title | Amoxicillin
Author | Paul Sullivan

ISBN | 979-12-22751-32-0

Youcanprint
Via Marco Biagi 6 - 73100 Lecce
www.youcanprint.it
info@youcanprint.it
Made by human

Table of Contents

Chapter 1

What is Amoxicillin?

This antibiotic finds application in the treatment of acute infections (not viral infections). Most commonly, amoxicillin is recommended to treat a variety of diseases, including sinus and chest infections, urinary system diseases, middle ear infections, and even some teeth infections. Prescriptions for amoxicillin may be given to you if your doctor determines that you have an increased risk of contracting an illness. Amoxicillin is a penicillin antibiotic, which cures infection by destroying the germs (bacteria) responsible for the ailment. Helicobacter pylori can be treated with amoxicillin. People with stomach ulcers are at a higher risk of contracting this infection. As a result, you will be prescribed other medications in addition to amoxicillin.

Type of medicine	A penicillin antibiotic
Used for	Infections (in adults and children)

Available as	Capsules, oral liquid medicine, soluble tablets, sachets of powder and injections

In 1972, scientists at Beecham Research Laboratories developed amoxicillin.

Because penicillin had such a restricted spectrum of antibacterial action, researchers began looking for penicillin derivatives that might cure a larger range ofillnesses. The discovery of ampicillin was a significantfirst step forward. Doctors could use ampicillin to treat a wider variety of infections, both gram-positive and gram-negative, than either of the original penicillin.

Amoxicillin, which has a longer half-life, was the outcome of in-depth studies. The benzene ring has an extra hydroxyl group, making it structurally distinct from ampicillin. Amoxicillin has a modest advantage over ampicillin in terms of solubility in lipids. As a result, amoxicillin may be able to eliminate germs slightly more quickly. Amoxicillin inhibits bacterial cell walls. It inhibits the cross-linking of linear peptidoglycan polymer chains, a key component of the cell walls of bacteria in both gram-positive and gram-negative conditions.

Amoxicillin was originally made accessible to the public in 1972, and it is now available in a wide variety of brands and formulations.

Chemical Structure

Name	CAS No.	Formula	Molecular Weight
Amoxicillin	26787-78-0	$C_{16}H_{19}N_3O_5S$	365.41 g/mol
Amoxicillin trihydrate	61336-70-7	$C_{16}H_{19}N_3O_5S.3H_2O$	419.45 g/mol
Amoxicillin sodium	34642-77-8	$C_{16}H_{18}N_3O_5S.Na$	387.39 g/mol

Physical Properties

The crystals of amoxicillin trihydrate were found to be orthorhombic in the space category P2, 2, 2, with four particles per unit cell, according to an X-ray diffraction analysis on a single crystal. The sulfur atom was out of the plane created by the other four atoms in the thiazolidine ring conformation. Hydrogen bonding between the p-OH group and acarboxylate of an adjacent molecule provides a new level of three-dimensional stiffness to the molecular packing and conformation of ampicillin trihydrate. An explanation for this may be that when amoxicillin trihydrate was dehydrated, it kept some crystallinity, as proven by X-ray powder diffractometry, and when water vapor is absorbed into it, it returned to the trihydrate. Amorphous hygroscopic material was formed when ampicillin trihydrate was dehydrated, and this amorphous substance continued to absorb water vapor long above the trihydrate threshold.

That's why, while comparing the crystal structures of amoxicillin trihydrate and ampicillin anhydrate, it was shown to be more stable because of the presence of the p-OH group. Because amoxicillin was unable to crystallize at the conditions utilized to make ampicillin anhydrate, this was a reasonable conclusion. An amoxicillin hygroscopic anhydrous crystalline monomethanolate was produced by solid-state elimination of the methanol. There is no remarkable notice in this last stage of the illness. When it comes to making amoxicillin sodium salt, most manufacturers use a powdery material. There are several ways to remove the solvent from various solvates, either in the solid state or by substituting a lower dielectric constant solvent in lieu of the solvent.

Melting Point

194 °C.

Chapter 2

What is Amoxicillin Used for?

Among the ailments amoxicillin can treat is bronchitis (infection of the bronchial tubes leading to the lungs), ear, nose, and throat (ENT), urinary tract (UT), and skin infections. H. pylori, a bacterium that causes ulcers, can also be eliminated in conjunction with other drugs. Penicillin-like antibiotics of which amoxicillin is a member are a subclass of antibiotics. By preventing the growth of germs, it is effective.

Amoxicillin won't help you get well by presence of viral infection like a simple cold.. The likelihood of developing an illness that is resistant to antibiotic therapy increases when you take antibiotics when you don't need them. This antibiotic finds application in the cure of diseases transmitted to humans by the bite of infected black-legged ticks and to avoid acute infection of Bacillus Anthracis also when skin is involved. Discuss with your medical practitioner before using this medicament.

Respiratory Tract Infections

Millions of people in the United States contact their family doctors each year due to upper respiratory tract illnesses. Antibiotics, while necessary in some circumstances, are often overprescribed. An overview of the correct use of antibiotics for ordinary upper respiratory infections is provided in this chapter. In patients with serious inflammation of eardrum, laryngeal cartilage, severe whooping cough, early antibiotic therapy may be warranted. Taking antibiotics may be necessary in situations of rhinosinusitis that have persisted past the point of observation. Patients with a cold or laryngitis should not be given antibiotics. It is important to use antibiotics in a judicious and evidence-based manner in order to keep costs down, avoid side effects, and drug resistance.

Doctors see a lot of patients with upper respiratory tract infections (URIs). An estimated loss of approximately 23 million working days is attributed to uncomplicated URIs in the USA each year. 1 Despite the fact that most of these illnesses are caused by viruses, antibiotics are used to treat a large proportion of them. Antibiotics were provided to 65 percent of patients in an important day hospital research of more than 50,000 Uniform Resource Identifier episodes.

Common Cold

A runny nose, a sore throat, a cough, sneezing, and nasal congestion are all symptoms of the common cold. Antibiotics have little effect on this diverse collection of viral infections. In the US, the general percentage of antibiotic usage for URIs diminished between 1991 and 1999. Broad-spectrum antibiotics,on the other hand, saw a surge in usage. An RCT comparing antibiotic treatment with a placebo in patients with acute URI symptoms lasting fewer than seven days, or acute purulent rhinitis symptoms lasting less than 10 days, was examined in research from 1966 to 2009. According to the authors, there was not enough evidence to encourage the assumption of Amoxicillin in childwood or adults with purulent or clear rhinitis.

Influenza

Viruses that cause influenza A or B produce an acute URI (upper respiratory infection). Patients of all ages are susceptible, although youngsters are most commonly affected. People over the age of 65 and infants under two years old are the most likely to die from flu. Preventive medicine relies heavily on vaccination. An antiviral medication regimen, Penicillin-like antibiotics, can shorten symptoms by a full one day if begun within the first 48 hours of symptoms developing. The use of amantadine as an influenza treatment is no longer recommended by ambulatories of safeguard.

Antivirals should be used to treat severe sickness, the elderly, children under the age of two, pregnant women, and those with chronic illnesses. Unless a secondary bacterial process is suspected, empiric antibiotic treatment should be discontinued once influenza has been identified. It's possible to tell if an antiviral regimen needs antibiotics by using Gram staining and cultures of bodily liquids.

Rhinosinusitis

There is an annual occurrence of roughly 13% in adults with acute rhinosinusitis in the outpatient environment. Purulent nasal release and obstruction face discomfort, decreased capacity in smelling, and severe cough are frequently noticed. 26 symptoms of rhinosinusitis can be classed as acute, sub acute, or chronic if they persist for more than 12 weeks.

Antibiotics would be overprescribed if all instances of rhinosinusitis were treated as if they were all bacterial or viral. To be certain that you have acute bacterial rhinosinusitis, wait at least 10 days following the start of your symptoms before consulting your doctor. Mucoid rhinorrhea, maxillary tooth or face ache, one-sided maxillary sinus soreness, and increasing symptoms after early recovery are more indicative of bacterial rhinosinusitis than viral rhinosinusitis.

If sufficient follow-up can be guaranteed, mild instances of acute bacterial rhinosinusitis can be handled with cautious waiting. Antibiotics should be started in these individuals if there are clear signs of worsening in a week time. Acute rhinosinusitis caused by bacteria must be treated with antibiotics.. Bacterial treatment for acute maxillary sinusitis provides a small statistical benefit over placebo in a Cochrane evaluation of primary care trials (n = 631 individuals). Because both groups had an elevate standard in cure, statistical relevance was ambiguous (89 percent in one side against 81 percent in the inactive substance group). When treating people with penicillin allergies, the first line of defense should be amoxicillin, although tri-methoprim/sulfamethoxazole (Bactrim, Septra) may be considered. If indications last for almost a week, a new antibiotic should be pre-scribed. No statistically significant difference was identified in the cure or improvement of symptomatology between long- and short-course antibiotics in an in-depth study with more than 4,000 patients. In individuals with severe bacterial rhinosinusitis, a therapy of only 5 or 6 days had the same success as longer assumption of antibiotic (more than a week).

Otitis Media

A recent beginning of signs, a secretory otitis media, are all neces-sary for the diagnosis of acute otitis media.

Haemophilus. I., Streptococcus P., and Moraxella C. are the most prevalent pathogens. The respiratory secretions of individuals with AOM have been shown to include viruses that may be responsible for many occurrences of antibiotic failure. Infants as young as eight weeks of age are at risk of contracting Streptococcus aga-lactiae, infection with Escherichia Coli and urinary infection in their middle ears.

AOM frequently resolves without antibiotic medication in children, according to cohort studies and RCTs. Important clinical research in the USA issued recommendations for the management of AOM in early 2000. To begin antibiotic treatment only in the event that symptoms continue or worsen, children older than six months are advised to follow these guidelines, which recommend monitoring instead. While this is true, two RCTs done in 2011 indicated that rapid antibiotic usage in children six to 35 months of age was more beneficial than observation in terms of outcomes. Diagnosis and follow-up were accomplished by the use of specific criteria, such as tympanometry or otoscopy. If a febrile newborn has AOM and is younger than eight weeks old, a thorough sepsis workup should be performed. If tympanocentesis is suspected, have the infants see an otolaryngologist. Children younger than two yearsold with bilateral AOM and others with AOM with earache should be given antibiotics immediately. The first-line therapy for AOM is amoxicillin (80 to 90 mg per kilogram per day, in two split doses). Amoxicillin should be started if the patient does not respond to the first course of antibiotics within 48 to 72 hours.

Rocephin is a second-line antibiotic that can be taken by kids who are regurgitating or have diarrhea. For the treatment of Acute Otitis Media, TMP and SMX such as erythrocin are ineffective. Antibiotics that are used for a longer period of time (greater than seven days) are less likely to fail. Clearance of tympanic membrane effusion in children with acute otitis media requires an evaluation in twelve weeks.

Tonsillitis and Pharyngitis

Pharyngitis is caused by a viral infection in around 90% of adults and 70% of children. Group A beta-hemolytic streptococcus is one of the most common causes of bacterial pharyngitis, if not the most common. In these circumstances, appropriate antibiotic therapy has been found to minimize the chance of rheumatic fever, relieve symptoms, and decrease the spread of the disease. In the case of glomerulonephritis, antibiotic therapy does not prevent it, and it has mixed outcomes in the case of peritonsillar abscess.

Prior to prescribing antibiotics, a test to identify the presence of GAS disease is strongly recommended. A more conservative approach is recommended by organizations like the American College of Physicians and American Academy of Family Physicians, which look at symptoms including fever, tonsillitis, lymphadenopathy in the anterior cervical region, and cough in addition to the standard Centor criteria. The risk of streptococcal infection is very low in individuals with a score of 1 or below, hence no additional diagnostic testing or treatment is recommended. Rapid antigen detection testing should be undertaken in individuals with a high risk, but additional variables must be addressed, such as contact with a person with proven bacteria disease. Streptococcal fast antigen detection tests should be conducted on persons who have a score of 2 or 3. Antibiotics are required in the event that tests show an infection. Patients with a range of risk of

4 or 5 should be given antibiotics.

Chapter 3

Warnings and Precautions: What You Need to Know Before Taking Amoxicillin

Consult your physician if your symptoms or those of your kid do not improve or worsen after a few days.

Anaphylaxis, a life-threatening allergic response, can occur as a result of taking this medication. Life-threatening anaphylaxis demands emergency medical intervention. After taking this prescription, if you or your child develops a skin rash, itchiness, shortness of breath or trouble breathing, difficulty swallowingor any swelling of the hands, face or mouth, contact your doctor immediately.

It's possible that amoxicillin can produce diarrhea,and this can be rather severe in some people. As soon as two months after stopping this drug, you can start feeling manifestations.If your child has diarrhea, seek medical advice before giving them any medication or administering any self-medication to them. Diarrhea drugs may worsen or extend the duration of diarrhea. In the event that you have any queries about this or if moderate diarrhea continues or worsens, you should consult your physician.

Doctors should be made aware that you or your kid are taking this medication before any medical tests are carried out. This medication has the potential to influence the outcomes of some tests.

Tooth discoloration may develop in certain young individuals who are taking this medication. It's possible that the teeth seem stained in various shades of brown, yellow, or gray. To keep your teeth clean on a regular basis or seeing a dentist p e r i o d i c a l l y will help avoid this. By assumption of this medicine, birth control may not be effective. Add another kind of birth control to your pill regimento prevent pregnancy. Condoms, diaphragms, and contraceptive foam or jellies are all examples of other forms. Make sure you talk to the physician before assumption of any supplementary medicine. Prescription and nonprescription (OTC) medicines, as well as plant-based and other supplementations, are comprehended.

You should not take Amoxicillin if you are sensitive to even one of the component of this medicine. Symptoms of this might be a rashes, as well as small bubbles of the neck. If any of the preceding conditions apply, do not take Amoxicillin. Any doubt you might have, ask your physician before taking Amoxicillin.

Precautions and Warnings

A consult is strongly recommended before taking Amoxicillin if you:

- Suffer from glandular fever (high temperature, pharyngody-nia, swollen lymph nodes, and heavy tiredness)
- Have an issue with kidneys
- Do not urinate frequently enough

Talk to your doctor or pharmacist before taking Amoxicillin if any of the above matches to you.

Tests of the Blood and Urine

In the event that you are experiencing:

- Glucose testing in the urine or liver function tests in the blood
- Tests for oestriol (used during pregnancy to check the baby is developing normally)
- If you're using Amoxicillin, tell your doctor or pharmacist

In addition to Amoxicillin, there are other Medications

Inform your doctor or pharmacist if you are now taking, have recently taken, or plan to soon take any additional medications or supplements.

- Allopurinol (for gout) may increase your risk of an adverse skin response if you take it with Amoxicillin. Your doctor may opt to change your Amoxicillin dose if you are on Probenecid (used to treat gout).

- If you're using anticoagulants like Warfarin, you may require additional blood tests. Amoxicillin might be less efficacious if you are utilizing other medicine simultaneously (such as tetracycline).
- Some medicines used by cancer disease and psoriasis) may increase the risk of negative results of Amoxicillin.

Before Using Amoxicillin

Consider the dangers and benefits of taking a drug before making your final decision, which is however up to your physician. Consider the following when taking this medicine:

Allergies

Be sure to tell your doctor if you've ever experienced a negative side effect from taking this or any other medication. It's also a positive intention to inform your physician if you have any additional allergies besides food. Non-prescription goods labels and packaging should be carefully studied.

Pediatric

Contemporary researches have shown that children's amoxicillin is safe and effective. A lower dose of this medication may be needed in newborns and babies 12 weeks of age or less who still have underdeveloped nephritic functioning.

Geriatric

As far as we know, no geriatric-specific difficulties exist that would make amoxicillin less effective for the elderly. Amoxicillin should be administered with extreme caution to older individuals due to the possibility of age-related renal issues.

Breastfeeding

Using this drug with breastfeeding has not been well studied in women. Prior to taking this medicine, evaluate benefits and dangers as well.

Drug-Drug Interactions

In certain circumstances, even if an interaction occurs, two separate drugs can be taken together despite the fact that they should not be used together. In such a circumstance, your physician might decide to adjust the dosage or take other measures to protect you. Your healthcare provider needs to know if you are taking any of the following medications while taking this medicine: The interactions listed below have been hand-picked for their potential importance, although they do not represent the whole range of possible interactions. Any of the following medications should not be used in conjunction with this medication; however, it may be necessary in some situations. Your doctor may alter the dosage or frequency of usage of one or both of the medications if they are given together.

- Chlortetracycline
- Cholera Vaccine, Live
- Demeclocycline
- Desogestrel
- Dienogest
- Doxycycline
- Drospirenone
- Eravacycline
- Estradiol
- Ethinyl Estradiol
- Ethynodiol
- Gestodene
- Levonorgestrel
- Lymecycline
- Meclocycline
- Mestranol
- Methacycline
- Methotrexate
- Minocycline
- Mycophenolate Mofetil
- Nomegestrol
- Norethindrone
- Norgestimate
- Norgestrel
- Omadacycline
- Oxytetracycline
- Rolitetracycline
- Sarecycline
- Sulfasalazine
- Tetracycline
- Tigecycline
- Venlafaxine
- Warfarin

Combining this medication with any of the following medications may raise the chance of certain adverse effects, but using both treatments may be the best therapy for you.

- Acenocoumarol
- Khat
- Probenecid

Other Interactions

Because of the potential for interaction, certain medications should not be taken with food or within two hours after consuming food. Taking some medications with alcohol or smoke might potentially lead to interactions. Discuss with your physician before taking your medicationto check possible interactions with foods, drinks or cigarettes.

Additional Health Concerns

If you have any other medical situation, this medication could not be the best choice for you. Check with your doctor if you have any other health issues, especially:

- Ceftin® or Keflex® should not be given to individuals who have an allergy to penicillins or cephalosporin antibiotics (e.g., cefaclor, cefadroxil, cephalexin, or Keflex®) or who have mononucleosis (viral infection).
- With severe kidney illness, use with care. As a result of the delayed elimination of the drug, the effects may be more pronounced.
- To make matters worse for people with phenylketonuria (PKU), the chewable pill includes phenylalanine.

Chapter 4

How Amoxicillin Works

Beta-lactams are a class of antibiotics that includes this one. Amoxicillin, inhibits bacterial cell work by connecting to proteins. Microbicidal killing takes place when the pathogens' cell walls are disaggregated, causing their dissolution.

When used orally, amoxicillin is stable in stomach acid and readily absorbed. Only the 400-mg and 875-mg forms of AMOXIL were tested when given at the beginning of a light meal to see if food affected the assimilation of amoxicillin from tablets and suspension.

3.5 mcg/mL-5.0 mcg/mL and 5.5 mcg/mL-7.5mcg/mL are the typical peak blood levels 1 to 2 hours following oral administration of amoxicillin capsules of 250 mg and 500 mg, respectively.

There was no difference in the peak blood levels of amoxicillin in the range of 1.5 to 3.0 mcg/mL after oral administration of the 125 mg/5 mL and 250 mg/5 mL suspensions, which were administered to 24 adult volunteers.

collected from individuals who fail triple treatment.

Quality Control

To verify the quality and precision of the sources utilized in the research as well as the methods used by the performers of the test control, standard susceptibility test protocols need the supervision of lab checkings. The following MIC range should be produced by standard amoxicillin powder, as shown in the table below.

Quality Control Microorganism	Minimum Inhibitory Concentrations (mcg/mL)	Disc Diffusion Zone Diameter (mm)
Streptococcus pneumoniae ATCC[b] 49619	0.03 to 0.12	....
Klebsiella pneumoniae ATCC 700603	> 128	—

[a] QC limits for testing *E. coli* 35218 when tested on Haemophilus Test Medium (HTM) are ≥ 256 mcg/mL for amoxicillin; testing amoxicillin may help to determine if the isolate has maintained its ability to produce betalactamase[4].
[b]ATCC = American Type Culture Collection

Chapter 5

Pharmacological Interactions Between Amoxicillin and Other Drugs

It is common practice to provide many medications to the same patient in order to treat both a single illness and a variety of illnesses. Inpatients often get many medications while in the hospital owing to a variety of comorbid conditions, such as cardiovascular, gastrointestinal, or neurological illnesses, skin problems, hepatic or renal impairment, or the irrational use of medications. The most prevalent cause of drug-drug interaction is dosage mistake, which can result in severe drug responses, and numerous pharmacological regimens.

Knowing whether or not co-administration of another medication therapy affects the efficacy and safety of one drug therapy is critical when it comes to drug-drug interactions. When the pharmacodynamics or pharmacokinetics of one medication are altered by the effects of another, we have a drug-drug interaction. One of the most dangerous kinds of medication interactions is the co-administration of two medicines. Various pharmacokinetic properties may be altered as a result of drug-drug interactions, according to published research.

Alteration in the absorption, distribution (dislocation from protein binding sites), metabolism (induction or inhibition of enzymes, etc.), and excretion of medications were shown to be the most prevalent evidences of alterations in the assimilation, delivery, metabolic rate, and elimination of chemical products. It's possible that certain medication interactions might lessen or improve the treatment efficacy and/or cause side effects. Identifying potential drug-drug interactions is critical to ensuring safe and effective treatment management.

Drug Interaction Table

Drug	Interaction
Aceclofenac	Amoxicillin's excretion rate can be reduced by Aceclofenac, resulting in a higher serum level.
Acemetacin	Amoxicillin's elimination rate can be reduced by Acemetacin, resulting in a higher serum level.
Acenocoumarol	Acenocoumarol's anticoagulant properties can be enhanced by Amoxicillin.
Acetaminophen	Amoxicillin's excretion rate may be slowed by acetaminophen, increasing the serum level.

Acetazolamide	It's possible that Acetazolamide can raise Amoxicillin's excretion rate, which might lead to a decrease in serum levels and a decrease in effectiveness.
Aspirin	Amoxicillin excretion can be reduced by ,resulting in an acetyl derivative of salicylic acid higher serum level.
Aclidinium	Aclidinium's elimination rate can be slowed by amoxicillin, resulting in a higher serum concentration.
Acrivastine	Acrivastine's elimination rate can be reduced by Amoxicillin, which might lead to a higher serum concentration.
Acyclovir	Amoxicillin's excretion rate may be slowed by acyclovir, increasing the serum concentration.
Adefovir dipivoxil	Amoxicillin excretion can be reduced by Adefovir dipivoxil, which might lead to a higher serum level.
Albutrepenonacog alfa	Albutrepenonacog alfa's elimination rate can be reduced by Amoxicillin, resulting in a higher serum level.

Alclofenac	It's possible that Alclofenac will lower Amoxicillin's excretion rate, increasing the drug's concentration in the blood.
Arsenic trioxide	This could lead to a higher blood level of Arsenic trioxide if Amoxicillin is used.
Atazanavir	Amoxicillin's excretion rate can be reduced by Atazanavir, resulting in a higher serum level.
Atomoxetine	Amoxicillin's elimination rate can be reduced by Atomoxetine, resulting in an increased fluid range.
Atracurium	Combining Atracurium with Amoxicillin can improve its therapeutic effectiveness.
Atracurium besylate	When used with Amoxicillin, Atracurium besylate's therapeutic effect may be enhanced.
Auranofin	Amoxicillin's elimination rate can be reduced by Auranofin bringing to an increased standard.
Aurothioglucose	Aurothioglucose's elimination rate can be slowed by amoxicillin, resulting in a higher serum concentration.

Azacitidine	As a result, the blood level of Amoxicillin can be elevated if Azacitidine is used.
Azathioprine	It is possible that Azathioprine can reduce the excretion rate of Amoxicillin, which might result in a higher serum level
Azelaic acid	Amoxicillin's excretion rate can be slowed by azelaic acid, resulting in a higher serum concentration.
Aztreonam	Aztreonam can reduce the elimination rate of Amoxicillin, resulting in a higher serum concentration.
Bacitracin	This could lead to a higher blood level of Amoxicillin if Bacitracin is used.
Baclofen	Amoxicillin's elimination rate can be slowed by Baclofen, resulting in a higher serum concentration.
Balsalazide	It's possible that Balsalazide willslow down Amoxicillin's excretion, increasing the serum concentration.
Baricitinib	Baricitinib's elimination rate can be slowed by amoxicillin, resulting in a higher serum concentration.

BCG vaccine	When Amoxicillin is taken in conjunction with BCG vaccination, the vaccine's therapeutic effectiveness is reduced.
Bendroflumethiazide	While Amoxicillin can be excreted more quickly with Bendroflumethiazide, the lower serum level and decreased effectiveness can be the outcome.
Benorilate	Amoxicillin's excretion rate can be slowed by benorilate, which could lead to an increase in the drug's serum concentration.
Benoxaprofen	Amoxicillin's excretion rate can be slowed by Benoxaprofen, increasing the serum concentration.
Benserazide	Benserazide's elimination rate can be slowed by amoxicillin, resulting in a higher serum concentration.
Benzatropine	Because benzatropine can reduce the excretion rate of Amoxicillin, the serum level may rise.
Benznidazole	Benznidazole's excretion rate can be slowed by amoxicillin, increasing the drug's concentration in the blood.

Benzthiazide	When using benzthiazide, Amoxicillin's excretion rate may increase, leading to a lower serum level and less effectiveness.
Benzydamine	Amoxicillin's elimination rate can be slowed by Benzydamine, resulting in a higher serum concentration.
Bepotastine	Bepotastine's elimination rate can be slowed by Amoxicillin, increasing the drug's concentration in the blood.
Bicisate	It is possible that Amoxicillin can reduce the excretion rate of Bicisate, which could lead to a higher serum concentration.
Bismuth subgallate	Bismuth subgallate can be excreted more slowly if amoxicillin is used, which could lead to a higher serum level.
Bisoprolol	This could lead to a higher serum level of Amoxicillin if Bisoprolol is used.
Bisoxatin	Bisoxatin's elimination rate can be reduced by Amoxicillin, resulting in a higher serum level.

Bleomycin	This could lead to an increased serum level of Amoxicillin if the excretion rate is reduced by Bleomycin.
Brivaracetam	Brivaracetam's elimination rate can be slowed by amoxicillin, resulting in a higher serum concentration.
Bromazepam	Bromazepam's excretion rate can be slowed by amoxicillin, increasing the drug's concentration in the blood.
Bromotheophylline	Amoxicillin's serum level could drop and its efficiency might be reduced if the excretion rate is sped up by Bromotheophylline.
Budesonide	Budesonide's excretion rate can be slowed by amoxicillin, increasing the drug's concentration in the blood.
Bumadizone	As a result, the blood level of Amoxicillin may be elevated if Bumadizone is used.
Bumetanide	Bacterial serum levels can be reduced by Bumetanide, resulting in a lower effectiveness of Amoxicillin.
Bupropion	Bupropion's excretion rate can be slowed by Amoxicillin, increasing the drug's concentration in the blood.

Buspirone	Amoxicillin's excretion rate can be slowed by Buspirone, which could lead to an elevated serum level.
Butabarbital	It is possible that butabarbital could reduce the excretion of Amoxicillin, which might lead to a higher serum level.
Canagliflozin	Amoxicillin's serum level could fall and its efficacy might be reduced if Canagliflozin rises its excretion rate.
Canrenoic acid	Amoxicillin's serum level could drop and its effectiveness might be reduced if the excretion rate is sped up by Canrenoic acid.
Captopril	Taking Captopril and Amoxicillin together may reduce the amount of Captopril excreted.
Carbidopa	Carbidopa can decrease the excretion rate of Amoxicillin which could result in a greater serum level.
Cefalotin	Cefalotin can decrease the excretion rate of Amoxicillin which could result in a greater serum level.
Cefapirin	Cefapirin can decrease the excretion rate of Amoxicillin which might result in a greater serum level.

Cefazolin	Cefazolin can decrease the excretion rate of Amoxicillin might could result in a greater serum level.
Cefditoren	Cefditoren can decrease the excretion rate of Amoxicillin which might result in a greater serum level.
Cefepime	Cefepime can decrease the excretion rate of Amoxicillin which might result in a greater serum level.
Dalfampridine	Amoxicillin can decrease the excretion rate of Dalfampridine which might result in a greater serum level.
Daptomycin	Daptomycin can decrease the excretion rate of Amoxicillin which might result in a greater serum level.
Deferiprone	Amoxicillin can decrease the excretion rate of Deferiprone which might result in a greater serum level.
Droxidopa	Amoxicillin can decrease the excretion rate of Droxidopa which might result in a greater serum level.
Duloxetine	Duloxetine can decrease the excretion rate of Amoxicillin which might result in a greater serum level.
Dyphylline	Dyphylline can decrease the excretion rate of Amoxicillin which might result in a greater serum level.

Edaravone	When used with Amoxicillin, Edaravone's excretion is reduced.
Edoxaban	Amoxicillin can decrease the excretion rate of Edoxaban which might result in a greater serum level.
Edrophonium	Edrophonium can decrease the excretion rate of Amoxicillin which might result in a greater serum level.
Enalaprilat	Amoxicillin can decrease the excretion rate of Enalaprilat which might result in a greater serum level.
Enoxacin	The serum concentration of Enoxacin may be increased when it is combined with Amoxicillin.
Enzalutamide	Amoxicillin can decrease the excretion rate of Enzalutamide which might result in a greater serum level.
Epoprostenol	Amoxicillin can decrease the excretion rate of Epoprostenol which might result in a greater serum level.
Etoricoxib	Etoricoxib can decrease the excretion rate of Amoxicillin which might result in a greater serum level.
Eucalyptus oil	Amoxicillin can decrease the excretion rate of Eucalyptus oil which might result in a greater serum level.

Ezogabine	Amoxicillin can decrease the excretion rate of Ezogabine which could might in a greater serum level.
Fenbufen	Fenbufen can decrease the excretion rate of Amoxicillin which mightresult in a greater serum level.
Gemifloxacin	The serum concentration of Gemifloxacin may be increased when it is matched with Amoxicillin.
Gentamicin	Gentamicin's elimination rate can be reduced by Amoxicillin.
Gestrinone	The therapeutic efficacy of Gestrinone may be decreased when used in combination with Amoxicillin.
Gimeracil	Amoxicillin can decrease the excretion rate of Gimeracil which might result in a greater serum level.
Givosiran	Givosiran can decrease the excretion rate of Amoxicillin which might result in a greater serum level.
Glipizide	Amoxicillin can decrease the excretion rate of Glipizide whichmight result in a greater serum level.
Glycerol phenylbutyrate	Amoxicillin can decrease the excretion rate of Glycerol phenylbutyrate which might result in a greater serum level.

Hydroflumethiazide	Hydroflumethiazide can increase the excretion rate of Amoxicillin which might result in a lower serum level and potentially a reduction in efficacy.
Hydromorphone	Hydromorphone can decrease the excretion rate of Amoxicillin which might result in a greater serum level.
Hydroxocobalamin	Hydroxocobalamin can decrease the excretion rate of Amoxicillin which might result in a greater serum level.
Hydroxyethyl Starch	Amoxicillin can decrease the excretion rate of Hydroxyethyl Starch which might result in a greater serum level.
Hydroxyprogesterone caproate	The therapeutic efficacy of Hydroxyprogesterone caproate may be decreased when used in combination with Amoxicillin.
Ibuprofen	Ibuprofen can decrease the excretion rate of Amoxicillin which might result in a greater serum level.
Ibutilide	Ibutilide can decrease the excretion rate of Amoxicillin which might result in a greater serum level.
Icatibant	Amoxicillin can decrease the excretion rate of Icatibant which might result in a greater serum level.

Icosapent	Icosapent can decrease the excretion rate of Amoxicillin which might result in a greater serum level.
Idarucizumab	Amoxicillin can decrease the excretion rate of Idarucizumab which might result in a greater serum level.
Idebenone	Amoxicillin can decrease the excretion rate of Idebenone which might result in a greater serum level.
Ifosfamide	Amoxicillin can decrease the excretion rate of Ifosfamide which might result in a greater serum level.
Imipramine	Imipramine can decrease the excretion rate of Amoxicillin which might result in a greater serum level.
Ketamine	Amoxicillin can decrease the excretion rate of Ketamine which might result in a greater serum level.
Ketazolam	Amoxicillin can decrease the excretion rate of Ketazolam which might result in a greater serum level.
Ketoprofen	Ketoprofen can decrease the excretion rate of Amoxicillin which might result in a greater serum level.
Ketorolac	Ketorolac can decrease the excretion rate of Amoxicillin which might result in a greater serum level.

Labetalol	Labetalol can decrease the excretion rate of Amoxicillin which mightresult in a greater serum level.
Mirabegron	Amoxicillin can decrease the excretion rate of Mirabegron which might result in a greater serum level.
Mivacurium	The therapeutic efficacy of Mivacurium may be increased when used in combination with Amoxicillin.
Moxifloxacin	The serum concentration of Moxifloxacin can be extended in combination with Amoxicillin.
Moxisylyte	Amoxicillin can decrease the excretion rate of Moxisylyte which might result in a greater serum level.
Muzolimine	Muzolimine can boost the elimination of Amoxicillin producing a decrease of fluid level
Mycophenolate mofetil	The serum concentration of Mycophenolate mofetil may be decreased when it is combined with Amoxicillin.
Mycophenolic acid	The serum concentration of Mycophenolic acid may be decreased when it is combined with Amoxicillin.

N-acetyltyrosine	Amoxicillin can decrease the excretion rate of N-acetyltyrosine which might result in a greater serum level.
Nabumetone	Nabumetone can decrease the excretion rate of Amoxicillin which might result in a greater serum level.
Nadolol	Amoxicillin can decrease the excretion rate of Nadolol which might result in a greater serum level.
Naldemedine	Amoxicillin can reduce Naldemedine's elimination rate, resulting in a higher serum concentration.
Nalidixic acid	The serum concentration of Nalidixicacid may be increased when it is combined with Amoxicillin.
Nalmefene	Amoxicillin can decrease the excretion rate of Nalmefene which might result in a greater serum level.
Naloxone	Amoxicillin can decrease the excretion rate of Naloxone which might result in a greater serum level.
Naproxen	Naproxen can decrease the excretion rate of Amoxicillin which might result in a greater serum level.

Nateglinide	Nateglinide can decrease the excretion rate of Amoxicillin which might result in a greater serum level.
Nedaplatin	Amoxicillin can decrease the excretion rate of Nedaplatin which might result in a greater serum level.
Nedocromil	Nedocromil can decrease the excretion rate of Amoxicillin which might result in a greater serum level.
Nefazodone	Amoxicillin can decrease the excretion rate of Nefazodone which might result in a greater serum level.
Oxazepam	Oxazepam can decrease the excretion rate of Amoxicillin which might result in a greater serum level.
Oxybenzone	Amoxicillin can decrease the excretion rate of Oxybenzone which might result in a greater serum level.
Oxyphenbutazone	Oxyphenbutazone can decrease the excretion rate of Amoxicillin which might result in a greater serum level.
Oxyquinoline	Amoxicillin can decrease the excretion rate of Oxyquinoline which might result in a greater serum level.
Oxytetracycline	Using Oxytetracycline in addition to Amoxicillin can reduce its therapeutic effectiveness.

Paliperidone	Amoxicillin can decrease the excretion rate of Paliperidone which might result in a greater serum level.
Palonosetron	Palonosetron can decrease the excretion rate of Amoxicillin which might result in a greater serum level.
Pamidronic acid	As a result, the blood level of Amoxicillin can be elevated when Pamidronic acid is used.
Pancuronium	The therapeutic efficacy of Pancuronium may be increased when used in combination with Amoxicillin.
Parecoxib	Parecoxib can decrease the excretion rate of Amoxicillin which might result in a greater serum level.
Paromomycin	The serum concentration ofParomomycin may be decreased when it is combined with Amoxicillin.
Patent Blue	Amoxicillin can decrease the excretion rate of Patent Blue which might result in a greater serum level.
Pefloxacin	The serum concentration of Pefloxacin may be increased when it is combined with Amoxicillin.

Quetiapine	Quetiapine's excretion rate cam be slowed by Amoxicillin, increasing the drug's concentration in the blood.
Quinethazone	Quinethazone may improve elimination range of Amoxicillin producing a decrease of fluid level with reduction of effectiveness
Quinidine	Amoxicillin can decrease the excretion rate of Quinidine which might result in a greater serum level.
Rabeprazole	Rabeprazole's excretion rate can be reduced by Amoxicillin, which could lead to a higher serum level.
Ramelteon	Ramelteon can decrease the excretion rate of Amoxicillin which might result in a greater serum level.
Ranitidine	Ranitidine can decrease the excretion rate of Amoxicillin which might result in a greater serum level.
Ranolazine	Ranolazine can decrease the excretion rate of Amoxicillin which might result in a greater serum level.
Rapacuronium	The therapeutic efficacy of Rapacuronium may be increased when used in combination with Amoxicillin.

Rasagiline	Amoxicillin can decrease the excretion rate of Rasagiline which might result in a greater serum level.
Reserpine	Reserpine can decrease the excretion rate of Amoxicillin which might result in a greater serum level.
Resorcinol	Amoxicillin can decrease the excretion rate of Resorcinol which might result in a greater serum level.
Ribavirin	Ribavirin can decrease the excretion rate of Amoxicillin which mightresult in a greater serum level.
Ribostamycin	Amoxicillin can decrease the excretion rate of Ribostamycin which might result in a greater serum level.
Rivaroxaban	Amoxicillin can decrease the excretion rate of Rivaroxaban which might result in a greater serum level.
Rizatriptan	Rizatriptan can decrease the excretion rate of Amoxicillin which might result in a greater serum level.
Rocuronium	The therapeutic efficacy of Rocuronium may be increased when used in combination with Amoxicillin.
Rofecoxib	Rofecoxib can decrease the excretion rate of Amoxicillin which might result in a greater serum level.

Roflumilast	Roflumilast's elimination rate can be slowed by amoxicillin, resulting in a higher serum concentration.
Rolitetracycline	When used with Rolitetracycline, Amoxicillin's therapeutic effectiveness may be reduced.
Ropivacaine	Ropivacaine can decrease the excretion rate of Amoxicillin which might result in a greater serum level.
Rosiglitazone	Rosiglitazone can decrease the excretion rate of Amoxicillin which might result in a greater serum level.
Rosoxacin	The serum concentration of Rosoxacin may be increased when it is combined with Amoxicillin.
Ruxolitinib	Ruxolitinib's elimination level can be reduced by Amoxicillin, producing an increased fluid rate
Sacubitril	Amoxicillin can decrease the excretion rate of Sacubitril which might result in a greater serum level.
Salbutamol	Salbutamol can decrease the excretion rate of Amoxicillin which might result in a greater serum level.
Trimetrexate	Amoxicillin can decrease the excretion rate of Trimetrexate which might result in a greater serum level.

Tropisetron	Amoxicillin can decrease the excretion rate of Tropisetron which might result in a greater serum level.
Trovafloxacin	The serum concentration of Trovafloxacin can be expanded in combination with Amoxicillin.
Tubocurarine	The therapeutic efficacy of Tubocurarine may be increased when used in combination with Amoxicillin.
Typhoid vaccine	The therapeutic efficacy of Typhoid vaccine may be decreased when used in combination with Amoxicillin.
Ulipristal	Using Ulipristal in conjunction with Amoxicillin can reduce its therapeutic effectiveness.
Vaborbactam	Amoxicillin can decrease the excretion rate of Vaborbactam which might result in a greater serum level.
Valaciclovir	Valaciclovir can decrease the excretion rate of Amoxicillin which might result in a greater serum level.
Valbenazine	Amoxicillin can decrease the excretion rate of Valbenazine which might result in a greater serum level.
Valdecoxib	Valdecoxib can decrease the excretion rate of Amoxicillin which might result in a greater serum level.

Valganciclovir	Amoxicillin can decrease the excretion rate of Valganciclovir which might result in a greater serum level.
Vancomycin	Vancomycin's excretion rate can be slowed by amoxicillin, increasing the drug's concentration in the blood.
Varenicline	Amoxicillin can decrease the excretion rate of Varenicline which might result in a greater serum level.
Vecuronium	The therapeutic efficacy of Vecuronium may be increased when used in combination with Amoxicillin.
Venlafaxine	Venlafaxine can decrease the excretion rate of Amoxicillin which might result in a greater serum level.
Verapamil	Verapamil can reduce the elimination rate of Amoxicillin, resulting in a higher serum concentration.
Vilanterol	Amoxicillin can decrease the excretion rate of Vilanterol which might result in a greater serum level.
Viloxazine	Viloxazine's elimination rate can be reduced by Amoxicillin, resulting ina higher serum level.

Vortioxetine	Amoxicillin can decrease the excretion rate of Vortioxetine which might result in a greater serum level.
Warfarin	Warfarin's elimination rate can be slowed by amoxicillin, which could lead to an increase in the drug's serum concentration.
Zalcitabine	The excretion of Zalcitabine may be decreased when combined with Amoxicillin.
Zaleplon	Zaleplon can decrease the excretion rate of Amoxicillin which might result in a greater serum level.
Zanamivir	Zanamivir can decrease the excretion rate of Amoxicillin which might result in a greater serum level.
Zidovudine	Combining Zidovudine with Amoxicillin may reduce its excretion.
Zonisamide	Zonisamide may boost the elimination level of Amoxicillin producing a decreased fluid rate with consequent inefficacy

Chapter 6

Dosage and Method of Application

Only take this medicine on advice of your physician in accordance to quantity prescribed. You can use it on an empty stomach or after eating; it does not make any difference.

For individuals who are taking the liquid medication orally:

- Shake properly before using and determine the correct dosage. This volume of liquid is probably too small for the typical home teaspoon.
- Oral liquids can be combined with a variety of cold beverages, including milk, fruit juice, water, ginger ale, and more. Make sure the youngster consumes all of the mixture as soon as possible.
- Continue to take this medication for the whole course of treatment in spite of good results you might have after the first doses. Otherwise, you might compromise the final result.

Dosing

The dosage of this medication will vary based on the patient's condition. Ask always your physician. Don't modify your dosage unless your doctor advises you to.

The strength of the drug determines the appropriate dosage. The time it takes to take the medication, the amount of dosages you should take each day, and the intervals between doses are all affected by the ailment you are treating with it.

Infections by Bacteria are Treated as Follows:

For all people weighing over 45 kilograms (kg) dosage is from 250/500 mgs three times a day, or 500/875 mgs twice a day, always at the same time.

If your child or newborn weighs less than 40 kilograms, the dosage must be set by your doctor and is dependent on the child or infant's weight. Every eight hours:

- A dosage of 20 to 40 milligrams per kilogram of body weight (mg/kg) is often administered, or a dose of 25 to 45 mg/kg/day, split and administered every 12 hours.

Ask your pediatrician the correct dosage for infants younger than three months. At 30 mg per kg of body weight divided into 12 equal doses, this is the recommended daily dosage.

Gonorrhea Treatment

One dosage of three grams (g) is recommended for adults, adolescents, and children who weigh 40 kilograms (kg) or more.

Children younger than 2 require a doctor-determined dosage. Probenecid (25 mg per kg of body weight) and methylprednisolone (50 mg per kg) are the most commonly prescribed dosages.

Use is not suggested for children under the age of two

H. pylori infection can be treated with the following medications:

Adults

- Every 8 hours for 14 days, the patient is given 1000 milligrams of amoxicillin and 30 milligrams of lansoprazole.
- A 14-day course of triple treatment with twice-daily dosing (every 12 hours) administration of 1000 mg amoxicillin, 500 mg clarithromycin, and 30 mg lansoprazole (twice daily).

Children

Your pediatrician will determine the dosage and time.

If The Dose Has Been Forgotten

Take it immediately when it comes up to your mind. Should it be very close to the next dose, simply omit the forgotten one and resume your usual dosing routine. Never take two doses together.

Chapter 7

Side Effects

A drug may have undesirable side effects in addition to its intended ones. Even if none of these adverse effects occurs, you must ask immediately for a physician's assistance. Medical treatment is rarely required for minor side effects. You may also want to talk to your doctor about strategies to avoid or minimize these adverse effects. Check with your doctor if any of the following side effects persist, are bothersome, or if you have any questions:

Common Amoxicillin Side Effects are:

- Nausea
- Vomiting
- Diarrhea
- Stomach ache
- Discomfort or leakage from the cervix
- Headache
- Rash
- Tongue that is swollen, black, or "hairy"

Amoxicillin can cause the following significant adverse effects as well:

- Clostridium spp. overpopulation in the intestines causescolitis.
- Fever
- Irritated and bloodshot eyes
- Inability to swallow
- A burning sensation on the skin
- Seizures
- Hives
- Red or watery diarrhea
- A rash that can be either red or purple, with blisters andpeeling skin
- Really painful stomach cramps
- Hepatitis B and C
- Swelling of the mouth or throat.

Chapter 8

Pregnancy and Breastfeeding

Amoxicillin is safe to take during pregnancy

Antibiotics of the penicillin class include amoxicillin. Only some antibiotics are acceptable during pregnancy.

According to the Food and Medicine Administration, amoxicillin belongs to B group medicines. This indicates it's okay to take it when you're expecting. Pregnant women who use amoxicillin may be at risk for birth abnormalities, according to the Food and Drug Administration (FDA). Amoxicillin did not cause any damage to growing newborns in animal experiments. If a pregnant woman takes this medication, it is considered minimal risk. Other antibiotics are also considered safe to consume during pregnancy by the medical community's expert panel. Clindamycin and erythromycin are two examples. There are additional medications in the same class asamoxicillin that are also included in this list. Pregnant women have to ask their gynecologist about the safest antibiotic to take in case of necessity.

Pregnancy and Amoxicillin Effects

After a few days of taking amoxicillin, you will begin to feel better.

It's strongly recommended to take the antibiotic following the indications given by your physician. Amoxicillin might improve your ailments right away; anyway, don't skip doses or stop taking it. Don't stop until you've completed your treatment plan. Your infection may come back if you don't take it as prescribed. Amoxicillin resistance might stem from this as well. This implies that if you get infected with something similar again in the future, the treatment may not work to cure it.

Amoxicillin's most prevalent adverse effects are as follows:

- ➢ Diarrhea
- ➢ Nausea
- ➢ Vomiting

Try taking this medication with meals and with a large glass of water if it causes you to feel nauseous. Amoxicillin might have more severe adverse effects on certain people. The sooner you notify your doctor of any serious side effects, the better. These are only a few examples:

- ➢ Responses to some allergens
- ➢ Hemorrhagic diarrhea, a lack of energy, and abnormal bleeding or bruises
- ➢ Discoloration of your skin or eyes, either visible or not

Diarrhea can be a serious side effect of antibiotics. Ask your physician straight away if you experience watery diarrhea or stomach cramps more than twice a day for at least two days. It's possible that you have a second infection, and this one might be harmful to your unborn child. This problem will need the use of a different antibiotic.

There are a number of Potential Dangers

A bacterial infection can become life-threatening if it isn't treated right away with suitable medications.

At any stage of pregnancy, amoxicillin is a safe drug with a very low-risk. Your doctor will determine if amoxicillin is the best option for you. This selection is based on the sort of infection you have and the length of time you will need to take antibiotics to treat it.

A lot of antibiotics can be dangerous during pregnancy, even if they are considered safe.

Pregnancy and Bacterial Illnesses

When you're pregnant, your own body shields your unborn child against a wide range of diseases. Among these are the common cold and the stomach flu. The placenta does not protect your unborn child from all types of illnesses, that's way your kid might become seriously ill in case of infection.

Birth deformities and respiratory issues can result from some illnesses, which can affect your baby's growth and development. Certain illnesses might also increase your risk of miscarriage or other pregnancy complications if left untreated. Ask immediately your physician if you have any doubt.

Breastfeeding when using Amoxicillin

Infections in neonates can be treated with amoxicillin, which is safe for nursing mothers to use. Breast milk contains amoxicillin, and while this is unlikely to cause harm to a breastfeeding baby, it might conceivably alter the newborn's natural flora. Taking amoxicillin with your newborn might cause diarrhea or oral thrush, which you should report to your doctor right away.

Chapter 9

BONUS CHAPTER: FREQUENTLY ASKED QUESTIONS

1. Which effects by intake of Amoxicillin without having introduced food?

Amoxicillin can be taken independently if you have eaten or not. Take this medication on a full stomach, unless differently advised, to avoid bad adverse reactions such as queasiness, cramping in the belly, and discomfort in the abdomen.

2. Can I take a double dose of Amoxicillin on the first day?

Every eight hours, a dosage of 20 to 40 milligramsper kilogram of body weight (mg/kg) is often administered, or a dose of 25 to 45 mg/kg/day, split and administered every 12 hours.

3. What is the appropriate Amoxicillin dosage for strep throat?

Dosages of antibiotics might differ based on a person's age and weight.

For persons who are not allergic to penicillin, the CDC recommends the following doses of antibiotics for strep throat. The dose regimen should be tailored to the patient's needs.

Oral Penicillin V

For ten days, 250 mg twice a day or 250 mg three times daily for children Adults and adolescents should take 250mg four times a day or 500mg twice a day for 10 days.

Oral Amoxicillin

Ten days: 50 mg/kg per day for children and adults (maximum 1000mg per day).

25 mg/kg twice daily (up to a maximum of 500mg twice daily) for ten days in children and adults.

4. Can you drink alcohol while taking Amoxicillin?

Yes, it is safe to take amoxicillin while drinking alcohol. Amoxicillin will not be affected by the presence of alcohol. The key is moderation. However, in order to give your body the best opportunity of fighting the illness, many medical professionals advise you to avoid alcohol.

5. Amoxicillin and paracetamolcan be taken in the same time? Possible Collateral Impact

You can take them together. Painkillers and antibiotics are safe to take in combination if you're not taking any other medications and are following the directions.

6. What can substitute Amoxicillin?

Cefdinir (Omnicef), cefpodoxime (Cefzil), and cefuroxime are appropriate substitutes for amoxicillin for those with moderate sensitivity (Ceftin). Amoxicillin-clavulanate (Augmentin) and these medicines are also routinely used as second or third line treatment.

7. Which is the Distinction between Amoxicillin and Penicillin?

Because it works on a broader range of bacteria, amoxicillin has an advantage over penicillin in terms of treating infections. Penicillin, which include both amoxicillin and penicillin, are a class of medicines.

8. What drugs can you not use while utilizing Amoxicillin?

Contrary to popular belief, you should not take these drugs at the same time. For further information, see a healthcare practitioner (e.g., a doctor or pharmacist).

> *ANTIMICROBIALS/LIVE TYPHOID VACCINE*

Toxic consequences can result from interactions between these drugs. For further information, see a healthcare practitioner (e.g., a doctor or pharmacist).

> *PENICILLINS/METHOTREXATE*

When used concurrently, these drugs may increase the chance of side effects. Ask for more details to your physician. SELECTED CEPHALOSPORINS & PENICILLINS/PROBENECID

> SELECTED PENICILLINS/SELECTED ANTICOAGULANTS (VIT K ANTAG)
> PENICILLINS/ORAL CONTRACEPTIVES

9. Is Amoxicillin safe?

Even though amoxicillin is a 100 percent safe and economical antibiotic, it isn't the appropriate choice for all illnesses. Antibiotics should not be shared with anybody. You are given an antibiotic that is tailored to your individual bacterial illness.

10. What occurs if you unintentionally take a double dose of Amoxicillin?

Amoxicillin is a time-dependent antibiotic. An increased dose will have no impact on bacteria, but will produce diarrhea and/or ab-dominal pain and discomfort as the most typical adverse effects.

11. Does Amoxicillin treat acne?

Research published in the International Journal of Women's Dermatology found amoxicillin to be useful in treating inflammatory acne, particularly in women with refractory illness.

12. Can Amoxicillin cause heartburn?

Another negative effect of antibiotics is that they might cause the stomach to become inflamed. The glands in the stomach release more acid when they are irritated. Heartburn can occur because of increased acid regurgitation to the esophagus.

13. How safe is it to take expired Amoxicillin?

Even if it hasn't gone bad, it may have lost part of its power by the time it reaches its expiration date. Even if it doesn't work as well against infection-causing microorganisms, it might aid in their development of resistance to the medicine. Because of this, the next time you require amoxicillin, it may have little or no impact.

14. Is a 3-day course of Amoxicillin enough?

As few as three days of therapy are possible for minor infections, but the normal course of treatment is five to ten days. When you get your amoxicillin prescription, you'll know how many days you have to take it. Don't worry if you miss a dosage.

15. Do I have to eat before taking Amoxicillin?

No, amoxicillin pills should be swallowed whole with a sip of water.

Never shatter or chew them. Amoxicillin is also available in drops
for people whocannot stand pills.

16. Why does Amoxicillin cause diarrhea?

It is common for people taking antibiotics to get diarrhea as a side effect.
Antibiotics might cause this side effect when they disrupt the normal
bacterial balance in the intestines. Some forms of dangerous bacteria
can thrive in this environment, resulting in stomach discomfort and
an increased risk of sickness.

Printed by Youcanprint

www.ingramcontent.com/pod-product-compliance
Lightning Source LLC
Chambersburg PA
CBHW052226150726
48002CB00003B/1293